BASKETBALL
SKILLS
FOR KIDS

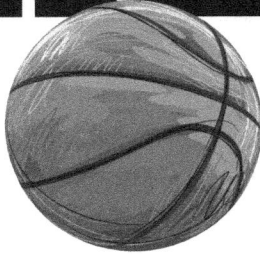

GARRY POWELL

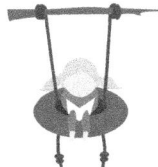

Wellington
books for kids

Basketball Skills for Kids

Author: Garry Powell
Illustrator: Randy Schrader
© 2022 Garry Powell

ISBN: 978-1-922872-22-7 (For paperback)
ISBN: 978-1-922872-23-4 (For digital online)

Wellington (Aust.) Pty Ltd
ABN 30 062 365 413
433 Wellington Street
Clifton Hill
VIC 3068

Love this book?
Visit kidzbookhub.com online to find more great titles.

Thanks to Matt, Luke and Scarlett for their help.

CONTENTS

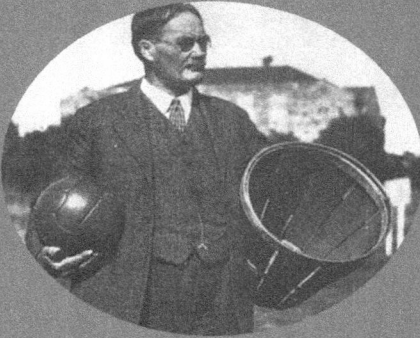
Dr James Naismith

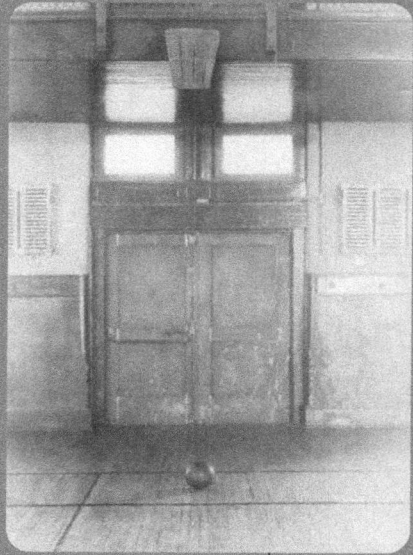
The first basketball court

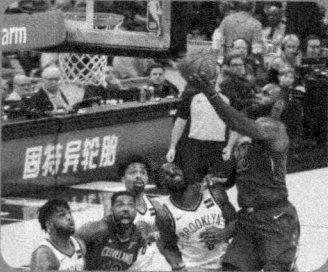
Le Bron James (above),
Michael Jordan (below),
NBA greats

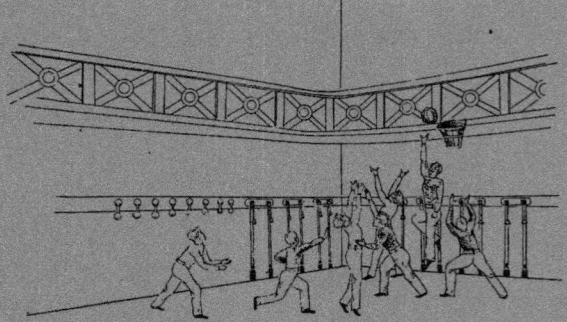

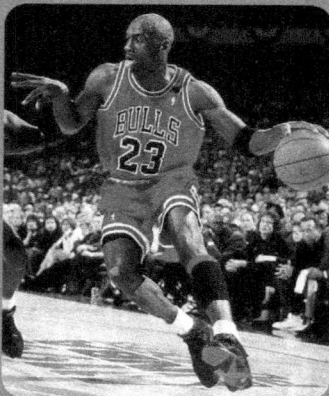

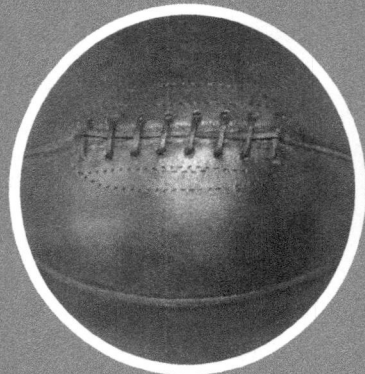
Early leather basketball

HISTORY OF THE GAME

This game originated in the USA in 1891 — Dr James Naismith from Canada developed it in a college in Springfield, Massachusetts that trained young men to become instructors at the newly formed YMCA. The game became popular as the students went on to teach around the country, and in 1939 it became an Olympic sport. It is now one of the most popular sports in the world.

Students in winter months needed an indoor game when they couldn't play outdoor games like soccer and football. Naismith first tried to adapt football and lacrosse for indoors, but needed it to be a non-contact game to avoid injuries. He called his game Basket Ball because goals were to be scored by throwing a soccer ball into peach baskets nailed to balcony at each end of the gymnasium. He added a backboard behind the baskets so students in the balcony could not knock away good shots from the opposing team.

BASKETBALL RULES

→ The aim of the game is to throw the ball through the hoop or ring (basket), which is each team's goal (10 feet high, with backboard). The team with the most points at the end of the playing time is the winner. The game is divided into halves or quarters, with the goal alternating. Timing, position and moves on the court are all important parts of the rules. The referee is in control of the game. Ask your coach to tell you about the rules of the game that apply to your team.

→ Five players per team are permitted on court at any one time. The team with possession of the ball is called the offence, while the team trying to stop them from scoring is called the defence. Once the ball crosses the mid-court line it cannot be taken back across this line. After each goal, possession of the ball is turned over to the opposition team.

→ Goals to points:
  * 1 point is gained from a goal scored from the free-throw line
  * 2 points for a goal shot from inside the 3-point line
  * 3 points for a goal shot from outside the 3-point line.

→ Moving the ball
  • The ball can only be moved by either dribbling (bouncing the ball with one hand) or passing the ball to a teammate. When dribbling stops, the ball must be passed to a teammate or used to shoot for goal.
  • A pivot is to have one foot grounded and to move the other foot when in possession of the ball. For a player to move with the ball they must either pivot or dribble.
  • The last touch out of bounds rule means the team that is not the last to touch the ball before it goes out of court gains possession of the ball in order to restart play with a throw.
→ Gaining possession of the ball can include:
  • stealing (taking the ball from the opponent or interrupting a dribble)
  • intercepting a pass
  • rebound (taking possession as the ball falls after a goal is missed).

→ Fouls

- Fouls that cause loss of possession, include physical contact, travelling (taking more than one step without bouncing the ball) and double dribbling (stopping then starting dribbling again). A player from the fouled team takes possession and throws from the side line).

- A foul deemed excessively rough (e.g. body contact) is called a technical foul, and can result in two free throws. After this possession continues with a pass-in from the side line.

- If a player is given five fouls they are sent from the court for the rest of the game and replaced with a substitute.

→ Time restrictions

- The offence must get the ball over the half-way (mid-court) line within 10 seconds. If not, the defence gets possession from the side line

- Players must not spend more than 3 seconds in the key or paint area.

- A limit applies to the time spent between gaining possession and shooting or passing.

- When a player stops dribbling, they must pass or shoot for goal within three seconds.

→ Free throws

- If a player has a foul against them while shooting for goal outside the 3-point line, then three free throws can be awarded.

- If a player is fouled while attempting a field goal, then two free throws can be awarded, taken from the free-throw line.

- If a player is fouled while shooting, but still scores, one free throw from the free-throw line can be awarded.

THE COURT

The basketball court is the playing surface, consisting of a rectangular floor, with haskets (hoops) at each end.

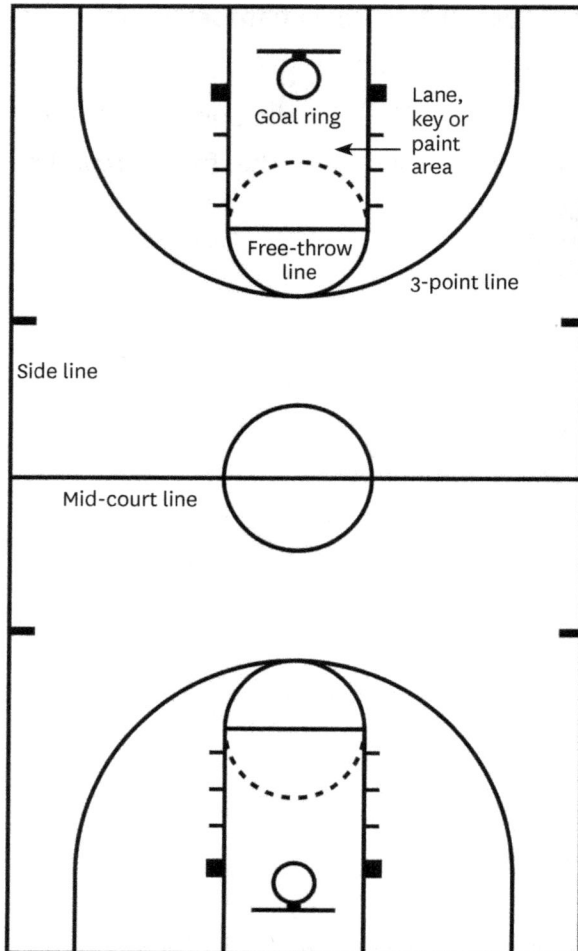

Goal ring

Lane, key or paint area

Free-throw line

3-point line

Side line

Mid-court line

SKILLS

Basic skills

Practice by yourself

Practice with a partner

Practice with three or more

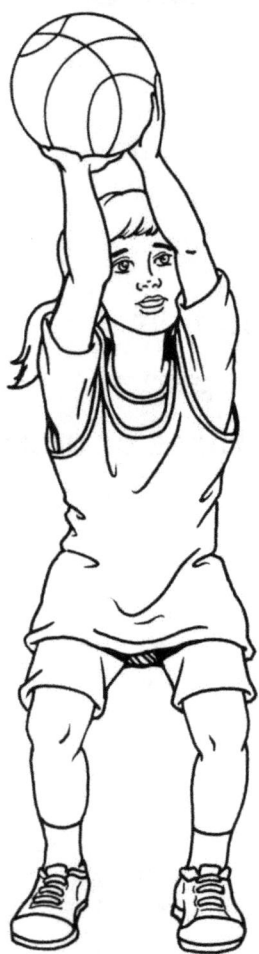

BASIC
SKILLS

TWO-HANDED THROW

→ This is used to pass the ball to a teammate.

→ A two-handed throw can also be used by very young players to shoot at goal.

→ Hold the ball in front of your chest — look at your target.

→ Hands are held at the back of the ball with about 60 per cent on the lower half — the same position as if catching the ball. Fingers should be evenly spread with the thumbs pointing towards the middle.

→ Step forwards and at the same time push the ball at the target with your arms straightening. The ball is released with a final flick of the fingers.

→ Your hands follow through towards the target.

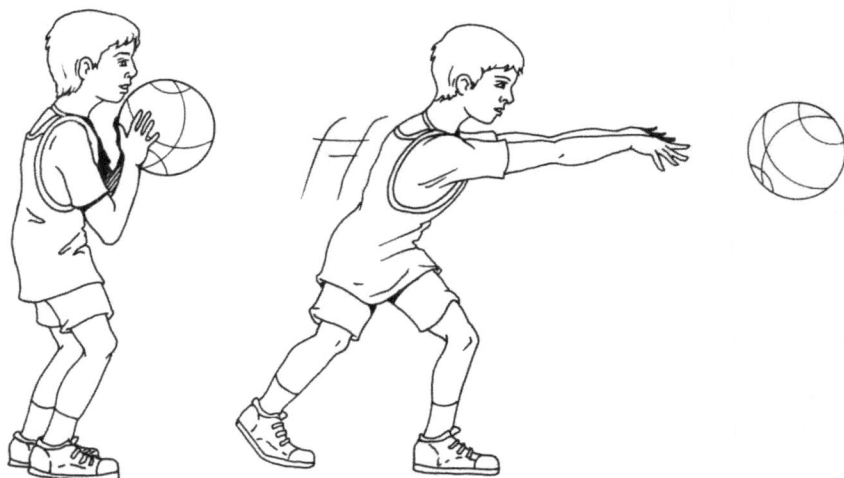

ONE-HANDED THROW

→ At first, the ball is held with both hands — the throwing hand is behind and under the ball; the other hand is on the inside of the ball to help hold it ready.

→ With the throwing hand the ball is taken back near your ear.

→ Step forwards on the foot opposite the throwing side (if throwing right handed, step with the left foot). At the same time push/fling the ball towards the target using your arm, shoulder and fingers.

→ Your throwing hand follows through towards the target.

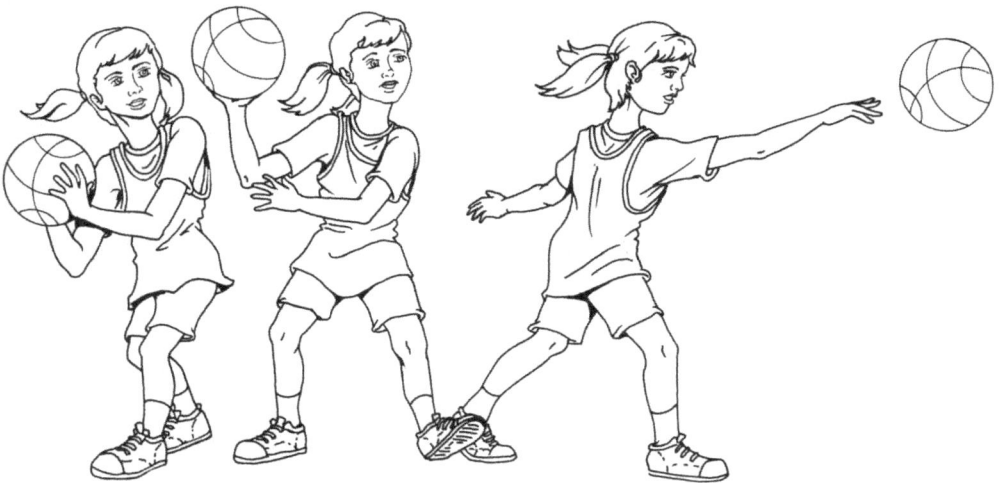

CATCHING

→ Watch the ball and anticipate when it will arrive.

→ Move your whole body to be in line and in front of the ball's flight path.

→ Both arms are stretched out in front, fingers spread, thumbs to the middle.

→ Watch the ball and track it all the way into the fingers.

→ To complete the catch, 'give' with the arms and 'hug' the ball near to your chest.

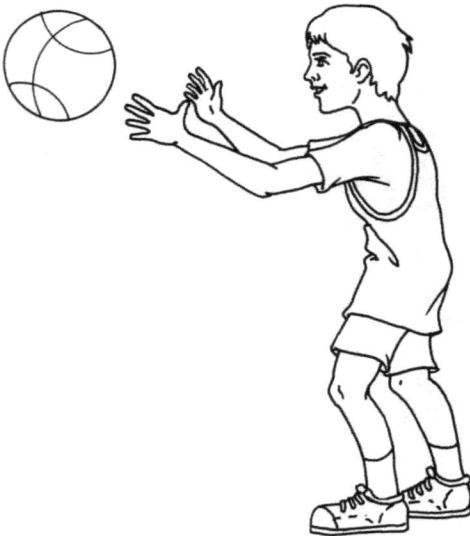

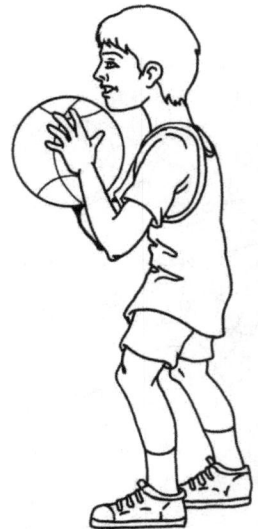

DRIBBLING

→ To dribble is to bounce the ball along without actually holding it. This allows the player to move with the ball. Only one hand can be used, and a travelling violation occurs when a player with possession of the ball takes a step without first dribbling

→ The hand is spread wide without tension. The fingers are spread over the ball and are used more than the palm of the hand for control.

→ The ball is pushed down (never slapped or patted) with relaxed fingers and wrist.

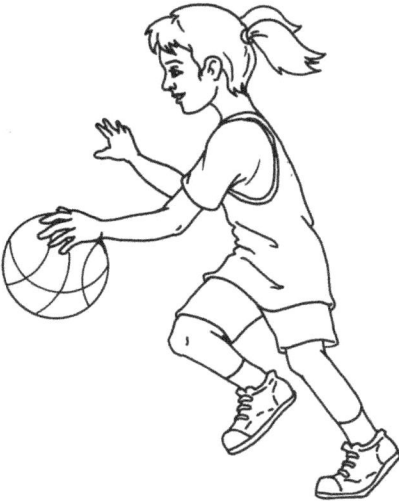

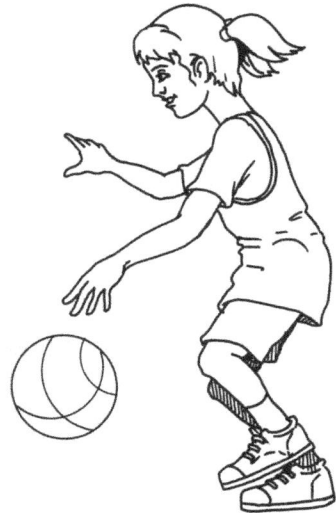

→ The body leans forwards towards the ball.

→ When the ball returns to comfortable reach, cushion it with the relaxed hand before pushing it back down again.

→ To help the dribble while moving forwards, the contact/catch on is slightly behind and to the side of the ball. The push should direct the ball slightly towards the direction of movement.

→ The body leans forwards towards the ball.

→ When the ball returns to comfortable reach, cushion it with the relaxed hand before pushing it back down again.

→ To help the dribble while moving forwards, the contact/catch on is slightly behind and to the side of the ball. The push should direct the ball slightly towards the direction of movement.

SHOOTING

→ This is to throw the ball so it passes through the basket as a goal.

→ Feet are comfortably apart with knees slightly bent.

→ The ball is held above the head with the strongest hand under and behind the ball. The other hand is used to 'steady' the ball.

→ Push with the legs through the body and arms to send the ball high towards the goal. The ball receives a final flick from the wrist and fingers of the throwing hand.

→ The ball should go in a high loop to lob through the basket.

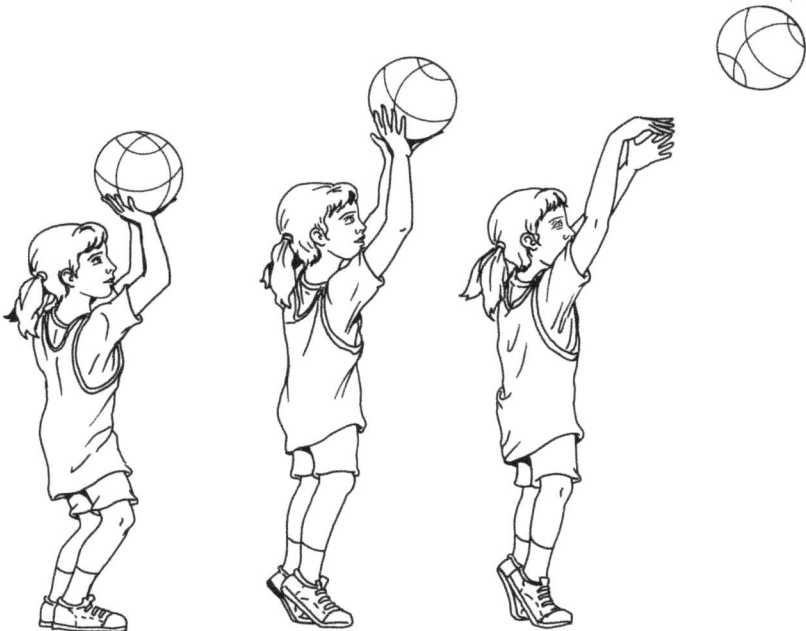

SKILLS PRACTICE BY YOURSELF

THROWING

→ Throw against a wall.

→ Throw to hit a target on the wall.

→ Increase the distance of the throw.

→ Throw at a marked target to score points.

→ Throw over an obstacle to hit a target.

→ Throw from different body positions.

All this should first be practised throwing with both (double) hands, then one hand (the dominant/preferred hand), then the non-preferred hand.

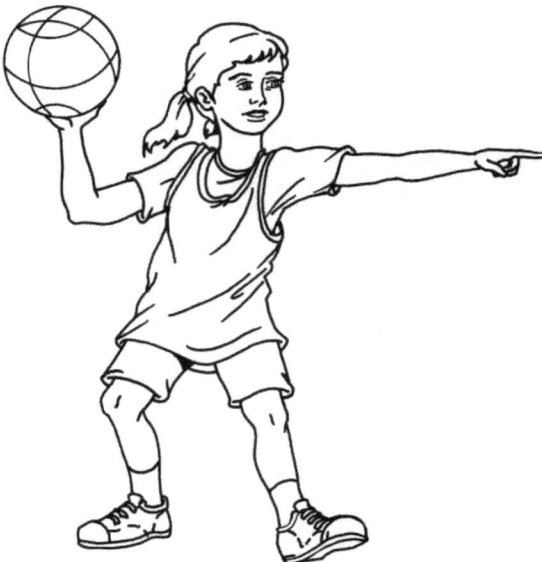

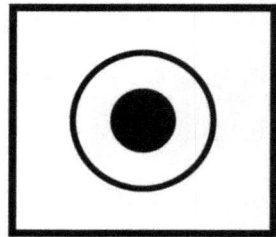

CATCHING PRACTICE

→ Throw the ball into the air and catch it.

- Throw into the air and clap hands once before the catch.
- Throw and clap as many times as you can before the catch.
- Catch the ball above your head.

→ Drop the ball and catch it.

- Bounce the ball and catch it.
- Bounce the ball so it goes high and catch it.
- Bounce the ball high and catch it above your head.
- Bounce high and catch in front of your chest.

→ Throw the ball against a wall and catch it.

- Let the ball bounce on the rebound before you catch it.
- Catch it on the full.
- Change the distance you stand away from the wall.
- Throw the ball on the ground so that it bounces up onto the wall and then catch the rebound.

→ Try to make as many repeats of each skill without dropping the ball.

DRIBBLING

→ Dribble (bounce the ball with one hand) while walking
- right hand only
- left hand only
- alternate hands: 4 with the right then 4 with the left without breaking the sequence
- 2 right then 2 left
- right–left, right–left, right–left, right–left.

→ High-bounce dribble: let the ball come to chest high.

→ Low-bounce dribble: only let the ball come knee high.

→ All the different dribbles while jogging, then running.

→ All the different dribbles going backwards, then sideways.

→ Dribble along a line.

→ Count the dribbles performed without making a mistake.

→ The walking set: 10 right hand + 10 left hand + 10 alternate hands + 10 high+ 10 low.

→ The complete set: the set of 50 different dribbles while walking + the 50 while jogging.

→ Rhythm dribbles — dribble in time to music.

→ Trick dribbles — between the legs, behind the back.

→ Record number of dribbles performed without a mistake: walking, jogging, standing still; right hand, left hand, alternate hands; moving — forwards, backwards, sideways, waist high, chest high, knee high.

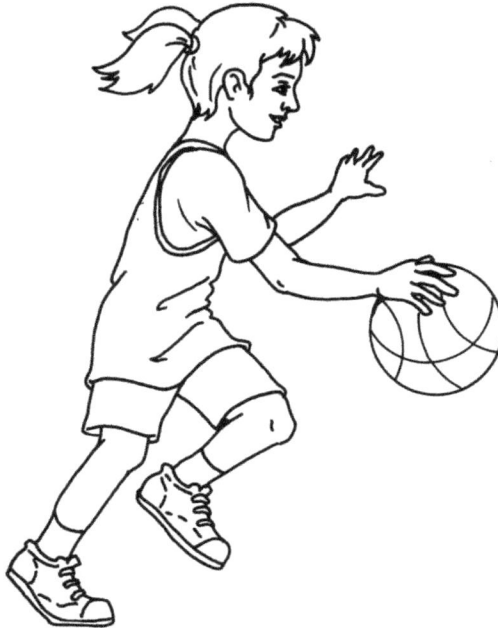

SHOOTING

Using a basketball hoop; a substitute ring, such as an old bike tube or tyre, a bin or drum; or even a mark on a wall.

→   Shoot hoops standing close to the basket

→   Vary the distance from the basket

→   Shoot using both hands, right hand only then left hand

→   Vary the angles from the basket

→   Shoot using the backboard every time

→   Layup practice — from standing, walking, dribbling

→   Jump shots using all of these variations

→   Shoot over and around a 'make-believe' opponent

→   Trick shots: underarm, bounce up, eyes shut, back to basket.

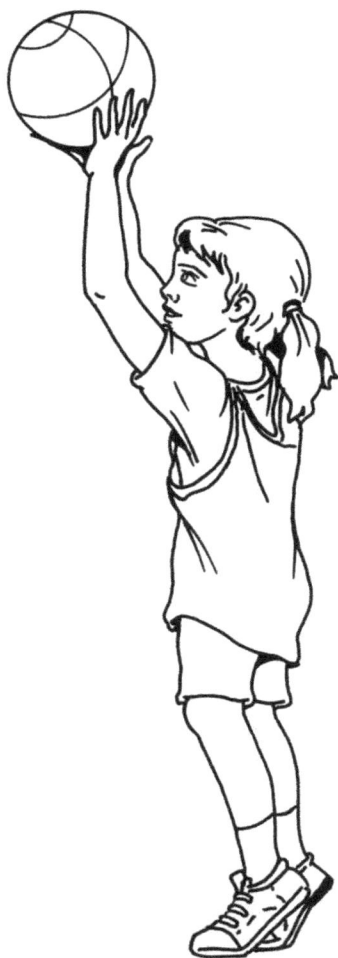

PRACTICE WITH A PARTNER

PASSING

When a throw is aimed so that the ball can be caught by a partner it is called a 'pass'.

→ Pass to a partner by throwing with two hands on the ball. Vary the distance of the throw, the height, the speed.

→ Pass using the right hand only — use all the variations (short, long, high, low, fast, slow, bounce, lob).

→ Pass using the left hand only.

→ Pass to a partner while moving and the partner is stationary.

→ Pass to a partner who is moving — the throw must be aimed at where the receiver will be when the ball arrives.

→ Pass when both the thrower and receiver are moving.

PROGRESSION BALL

→ Partners are an equal distance from a midline.

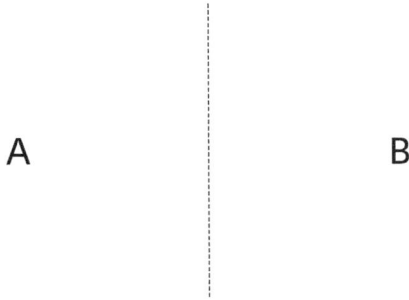

A   B

→ Partner A throws the ball to partner B. If B catches the ball, they take one step backwards. If the throw/pass is not within the reach of B, then A has to take a step forwards.

→ Partner B then throws to A from their new starting position.

→ The contest winner is the player furthest from the midline after an equal nominated number of passes.

FORCE BACK

→ Partners are an equal distance from a midline.

A | B

→ Partner A throws the ball towards partner B — this pass must have a landing point within 2 metres of B. If B catches the ball, they then throw the ball back towards A from exactly where it was caught. If the ball is not caught, B takes a step backwards along the throw line and A takes a step forwards along the throw line. These positions now become their pass and catch points.

→ The aim of this game is to force the partner back until they can catch the return throw on the opposite side of the midline from where they started.

REBOUND BALL

→ Player A throws the ball at a wall and player B has to catch the return ball 'on the full' or after one bounce. The throw can be varied by: distance, height on the wall, bounce pass.

→ After ten successful catches the partners change roles.

GOAL BALL

→ Player A tries to throw the ball through player B's goal — player B defends their goal.

→ The winner is the player with the most goals after 10 throws each. Variations can be made by changing the size of the goal area or the distance thrown.

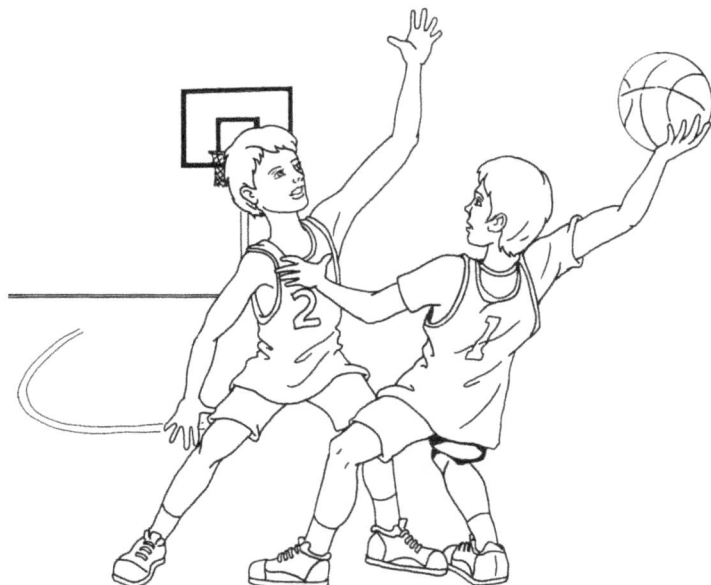

CATCHING PRACTICE

→ All the passing practices also involve catching.

→ Catch the ball at stomach height, chest height, overhead.

→ Catch a ball kicked by a partner.

→ Catch a ball as it rebounds from a wall.

→ Catch a ball as it rebounds from the backboard or basket.

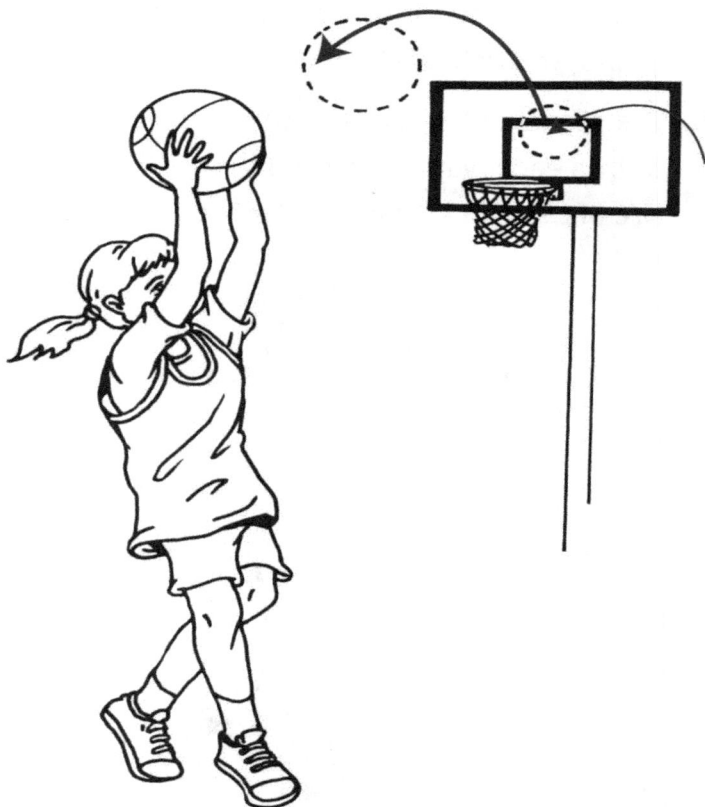

DRIBBLING

→ **Follow the Leader** — partners take it in turns to lead. The leader does a type of dribble activity which the follower must copy:

- using right hand only
- using left hand only
- using alternate hands (e.g. five with the right followed by five with the left)
- different heights and speed of bounce
- while moving differently — walking, jogging, running, backwards, sideways.

→ **Mirroring** — this is a more difficult form of follow the leader. The follower has to have their ball moving exactly the same as the leader at exactly the same time — as if looking into a mirror.

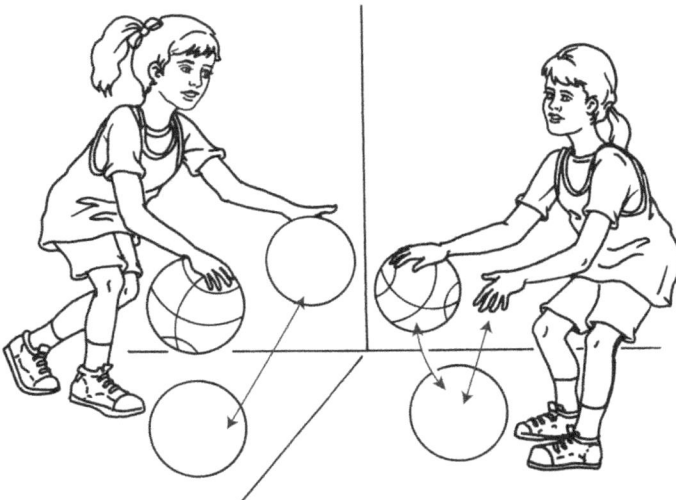

→ Joined dribbling — partners stand side by side and join inside hands, then dribble variations with the outside hands.

→ Races — dribble race a partner in a set method over a set distance.

→ Partner tag — while dribbling the ball one tries to tag the other. Take turns at being 'IT'.

SHOOTING

→ **Follow the Leader** — partners take it in tum to lead. The leader does a type of shot that the follower must copy:

- right hand
- left hand
- both hands
- off the back board
- basket only
- from dribbling

→ **Around the Clock** — Partners take turns to shoot from the 9 o'clock to 3 o'clock positions. What is the best score from these seven positions?

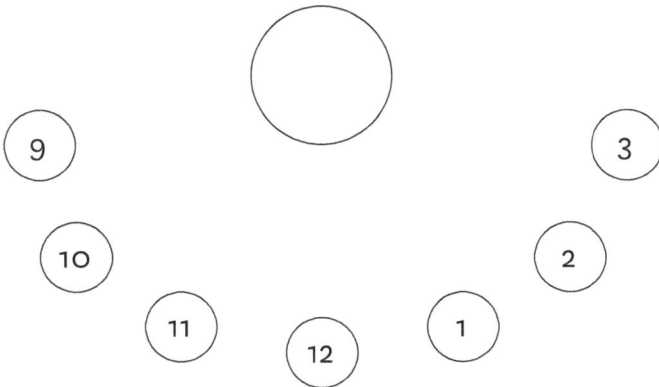

→ **10 up or 20 up**

- Take it in turns to shoot from different positions, changing angles and distance. After an equal number of shots from each position — whoever gets to target or end number of goals first is the winner.

→ **Rebound**

- One partner shoots. The other catches the rebound no matter if it is a goal or not and then shoots from the spot where the ball is caught.

→ **One on one**

- One partner shoots over a partner's defence — arm or arms. Shooting varies: over, around, past, in front, from dribbling.

PRACTICE WITH THREE OR MORE

DRIBBLE

→ **Relays**

- Starting from behind a line, each member of the group/class/team dribbles the ball across an opposite line and returns.

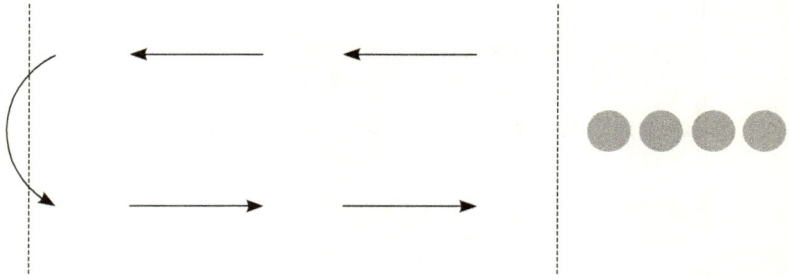

- Dribble around an obstacle course.

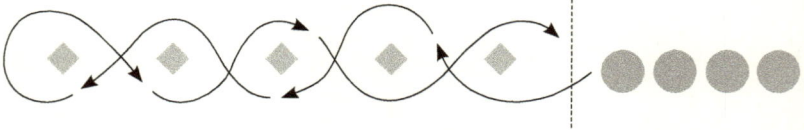

- Dribble to a wall — pass the ball at the wall — catch and return.

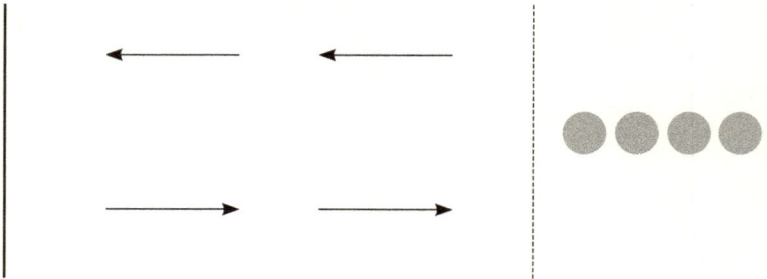

→ **Dribble Spry**

* The leader (No.1) throws the ball to No. 2 who catches it. No. 2 then runs and dribbles behind the group to take the place of the leader.

* The leader moves into position 2 and all players move up one place. Player No. 2 is now the leader and now passes the ball to No. 3 who is in their old position 2. Player 3 now dribbles the ball behind the group and out to the front to be the new leader — and so on.

* This process continues until all players are back in their original starting positions.

PASS AND CATCH

→ **Interception in Threes**

* Numbers 1 and 3 make as many passes to each other without No. 2 intercepting.

(1)   (2)   (3)

→ **Ten Trips**

- The three players are 3–4 metres apart.
- Number 1 throws to No. 3 who passes to No. 2 who in turn passes to No. l. That circuit is one trip. This process continues until there are ten trips.
- The three players then rotate position.
- This practice can be made more difficult by ruling that if the ball is not caught then that trip cannot be counted in the total.

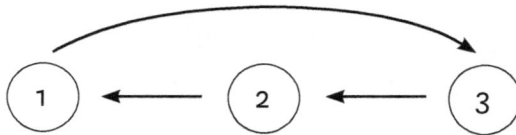

→ **Corner Spry**

- The leader (No. 1) throws the ball and receives it back from players 2–6. The last player in the line (No. 6) runs with the ball to the leader's position.
- At the same time all players move one place to their right and the leader replaces No. 2 in the line.
- This movement continues until all players have been leader.

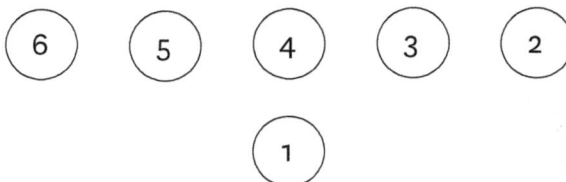

→ **Circle Pass**

- In a circle formation, the centre player (No. 1) passes the ball and receives back in order to players 2–6.
- Each player takes a turn to be the centre.

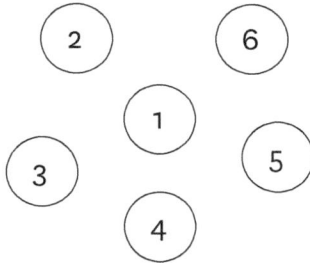

→ **In and Out**

- In a circle formation, the centre player (No. 1) passes the ball and receives back in order to players 2–6. On receiving the ball No. 6 runs to the centre and becomes the leader while the first leader replaces them in the circle (swap positions).
- The new centre leader's first pass and receive will be to the player who replaced them in the circle.
- This process is repeated until all players have had a turn in the centre.

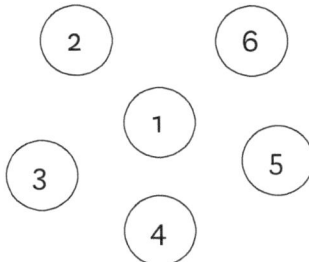

→ **Bob Ball**

- Players in a line, all facing the same line direction (looking at the back of the player in front of them). The leader (No. 1) is 2 metres in front of the first in line.

- The leader passes the ball and receives in tum from the first in line (No. 2). No. 2 on returning the ball to the leader bobs down on their spot. The leader then passes over the bobbed person to the next in line.

- This process continues until each player has received and returned.

→ A game can be made of this practice by the leader passing and receiving in front order and the reverse order:

- Leader to 2, 3, 4, 5, 4, 3, 2. On receiving the ball on its return rotation, No. 2 keeps the ball, runs around the line of players and replaces the leader.

- The initial leader replaces the runner on their spot and the process continues until all players have been to the front to be leader.

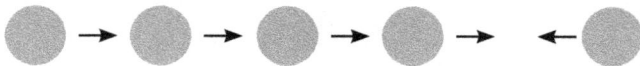

→ **Cross Ball**

  + Players are spaced alternately 3 metres apart.

  + Number 1 passes to No. 2, then 2–3, 3–4, 4–5, 5–6, 6–7, 7–8, 8–9, 9–10.

  + Then the passing returns along the line: 8–7, 7–6, etc. The practice ends when the ball is back with No. 1.

→ To increase the difficulty of this practice, the number of times the ball completes this circuit can be increased and the sequence timed.

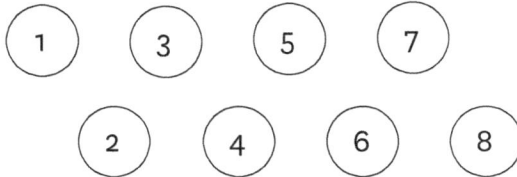

SHOOTING

Shooting practices for a group are much the same as for pairs.

→ **Follow the Leader**

- Players take it in turns to be leader.
- The leader does a type of shot that all followers must copy. This can be: right hand, left hand, both hands, basket only, backboard only, layup from dribbling.

→ **School Day Clock**

- The first player shoots from the 9 o'clock position, then 10 o'clock, 11, 12, 1, 2, 3.
- Each player follows this procedure.

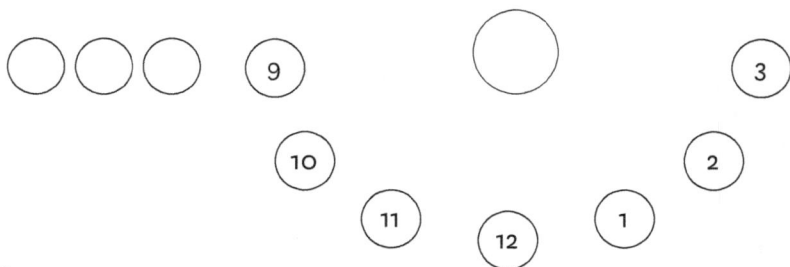

→ **10 Up**

- Players take turns from nominated set positions — changing angles and distance to increase the difficulty.
- After an equal number of shots, whoever gets 10 goals first is the winner.

DIFFERENT GAMES

→ End Ball

- This game needs a playing area of between 12m × 6m and 24m × 12m. This is then divided into two end zones and two team zones.

- The two teams of equal numbers both have a goal area where they have three players acting as catchers and a playing area in which they can move freely without the ball, but not enter the oppositions playing area.

- The game is started by a 'tip off' or 'throw up' at the centre circle. The team winning possession of the ball then can pass the ball between themselves with the aim of getting into a position where they can lob the ball over their opponents to be caught by one of their own catchers.

- Players cannot run with the ball.

- If the ball is intercepted the other team attempts to get the ball to their catchers. If the ball goes out of bounds the team loses possession.

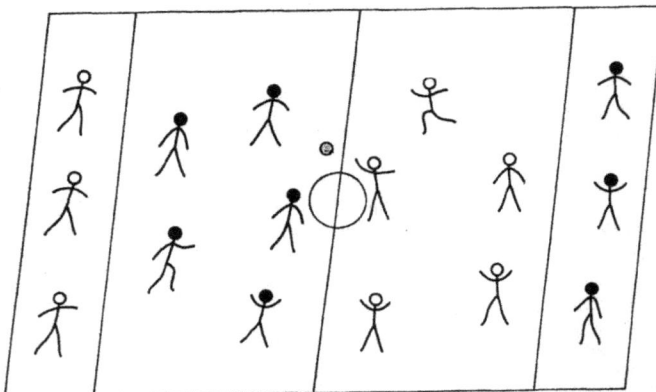

→ **Corner Ball**

- The game is started by a basketball style 'tip off' in the centre circle. Players then pass the ball but cannot run with it.

- Players attempt to pass the ball to their team mates to score a goal. If the ball goes out of bounds, the last touch rule applies (the last team to touch the ball before it goes out loses possession). The other team restarts play with a throw from the sideline.

- After each goal, play is restarted with a centre 'tip off'.

- As skills develop, this game can be played with dribbling allowed to enable players to move with the ball.

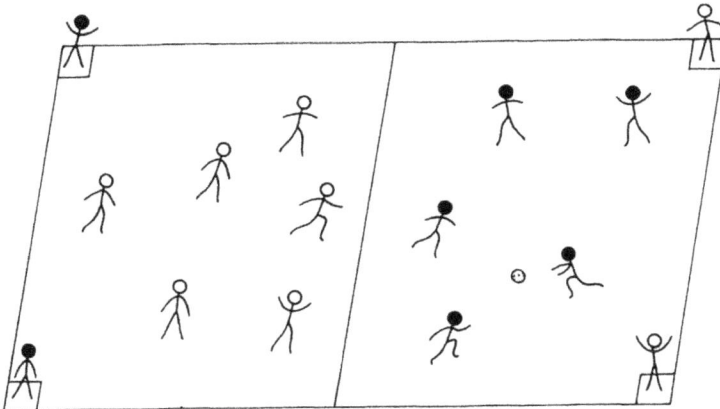

→ Invaders

- The playing area is dived into halves — players are positioned in these opposite halves.
- One player from each team is sent into the opposition area to be the 'invader'.
- The aim of the game is to get the ball to the invader in the opposition's half. When a successful pass has been made to an invader, an additional invader also goes into that half.
- Scoring starts only when three invaders are in an opponent's half. Points are then scored for each successful pass to an invader.
- Passing rules are as for basketball.

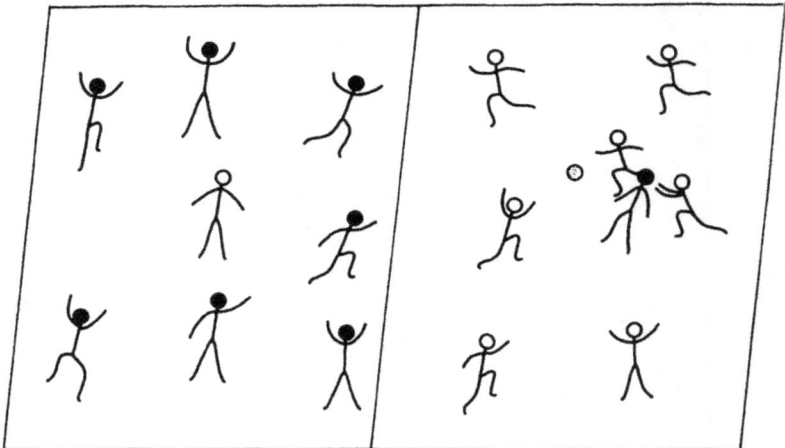

→ **Permit Ball**

- The game is started by a pass from the permit area.
- Players then pass the ball until they are able to pass it to their goalie, who is then allowed to shoot for a goal.
- If the ball is intercepted, two of the intercepting team become the permit and goal players and they begin a new attack.
- The rules are as for basketball but without the dribbling that allows players to move when in possession of the ball.

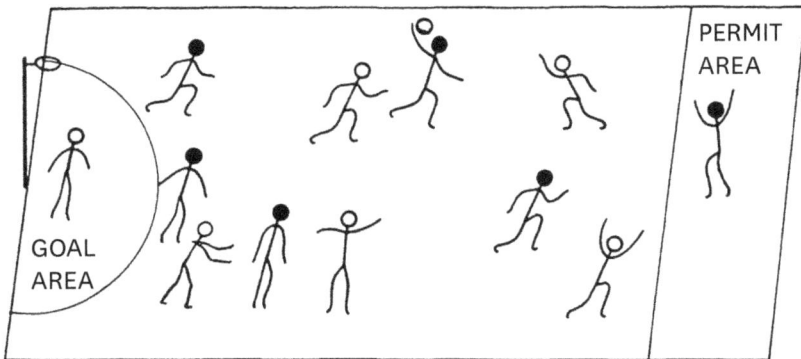

→ Mat Ball

- Equal teams of 3–5.
- Using dribbling and passing as in basketball, teams try to get the ball to their goalie who is standing on a mat. This scores one point. The goalie is not allowed off the mat and no one else is allowed on it.

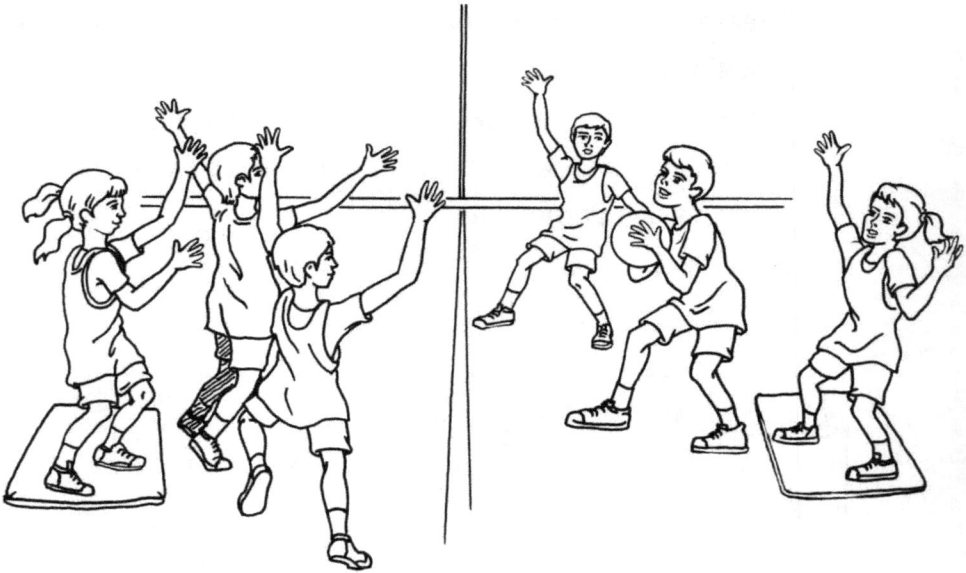

→ **One on One, Two on Two or Three on Three played on a half of a basketball court.**

- ♦ This game is played team on team, whether it be one on one, two on two, three on three.

- ♦ Team A starts with the ball and faces Team B. Team A can shoot immediately or dribble to position and shoot while Team B defends. After each attempt the opposite team starts with the ball.

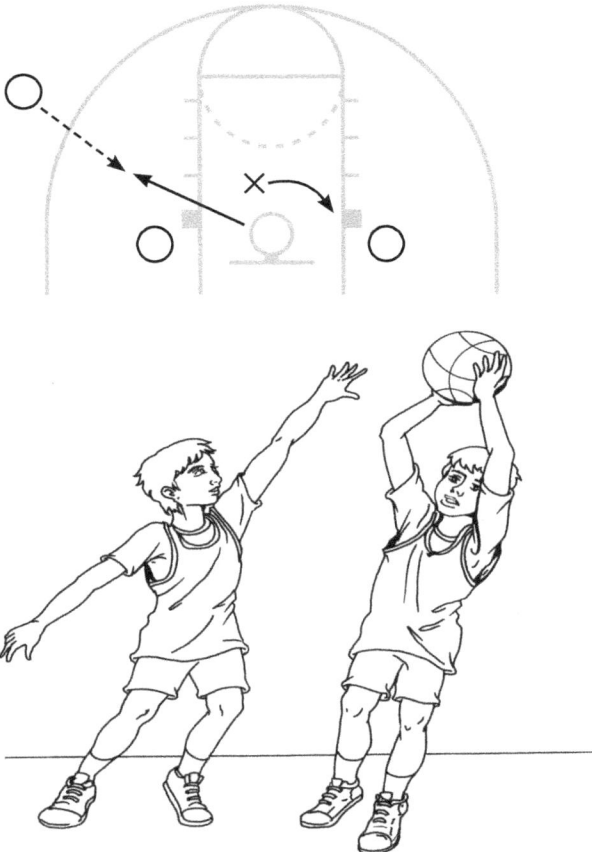

WARM UP AND WARM DOWN

→ **Jogging**

- on the spot
- slow runs forwards
- slow runs backwards

→ **Neck and shoulders**

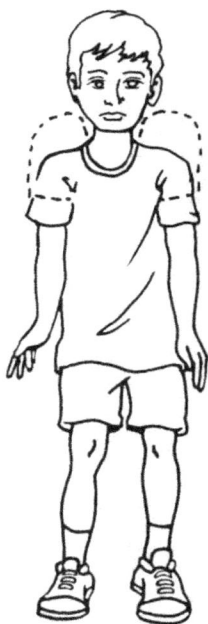

- Stand with feet shoulder width apart, shrug shoulders near to ears — left, right, both.

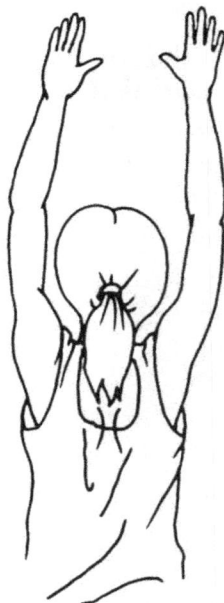

- With arms raised, move shoulder blades closer together.

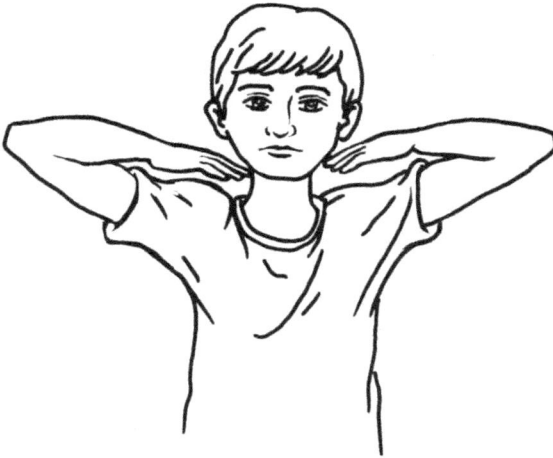

- With fingers touching the neck, elbows pressed back — rotate the elbows forwards and then backwards — left, right, both.

- With fingers interlaced, palms down, back straight — press hands downwards for the count of four; then with hands above head and palms up, press upwards for the count of four.

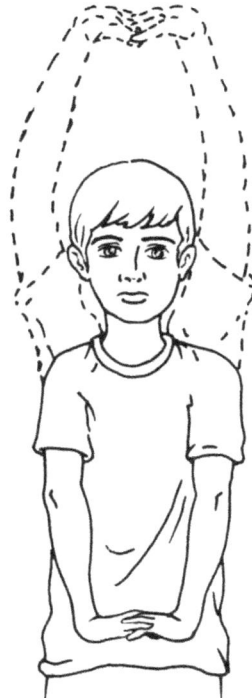

→ **Trunk and arms**

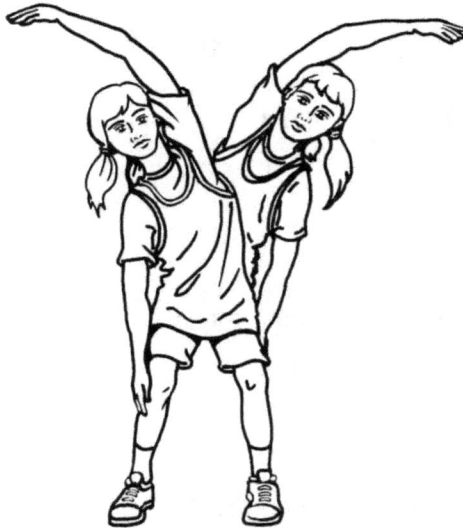

♦ Side stretching — feet shoulder width apart, one arm held high with palm inwards; opposite arm held down with palm along thigh: bend the trunk slowly sidewards to slide palm down the leg, then return to vertical. Repeat to opposite side with a change of arms — left, right alternate.

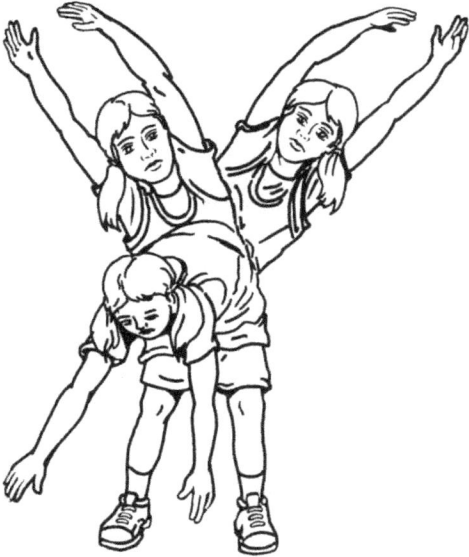

- Trunk circling — with arms above head, circle arms to the right in slow sweeping movements with hands passing low, at least at knee level.
- Repeat to the left, then alternate.

- Arm circles — with arms straight, and standing erect, make arm circles — right arm, left arm, both arms alternate. First done swinging forwards and then backwards.

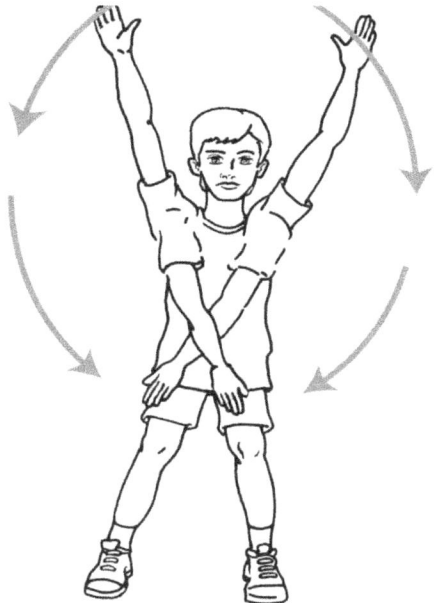

→ **Legs and back**

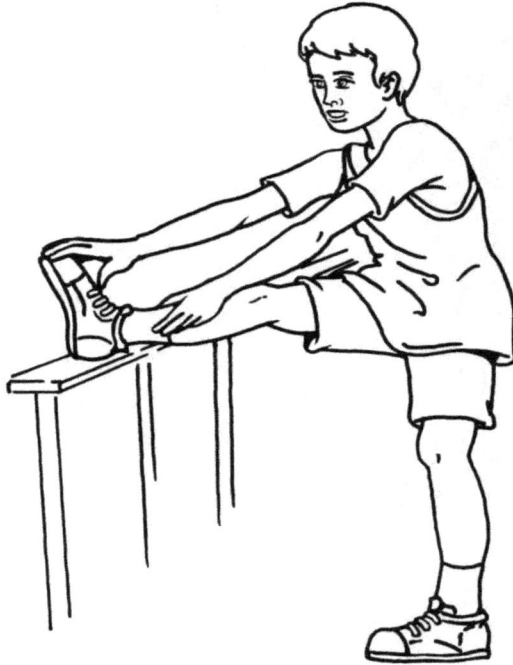

* Hamstring stretch — one leg with heel placed on support between knee and groin high, toe pointing up. Lean the body gently forwards until a slight stretch can be felt in the hamstring. This position is held for 5–10 seconds then the body returns to the start position. This is repeated 5–10 times and then same process for the other leg.

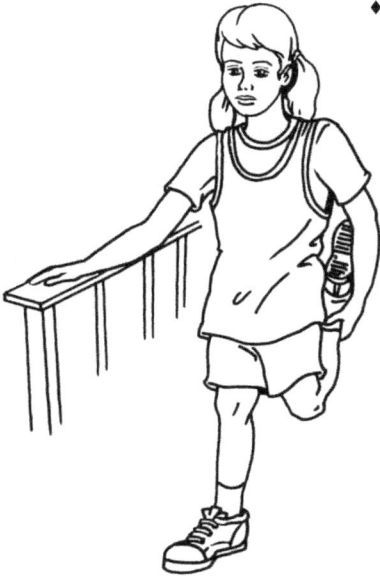

• Quadriceps stretch — one hand holding a support, and standing on one leg (the same side as the support arm). The opposite foot is held near the ankle and then the foot is gently pulled towards the buttock until a slight stretch is felt. This position is held for 5–10 seconds then returns to the starting position and then the same process for the other leg.

• Calf stretch — facing a wall and with palms against it. Put one foot in front of the other, front knee slightly bent and back knee straight but with the heel on the ground. The front knee is gently bent further until a slight stretch can be felt in the calf of the back leg. Hold for 5–10 seconds with 5–10 repetitions, then repeat using the other leg.

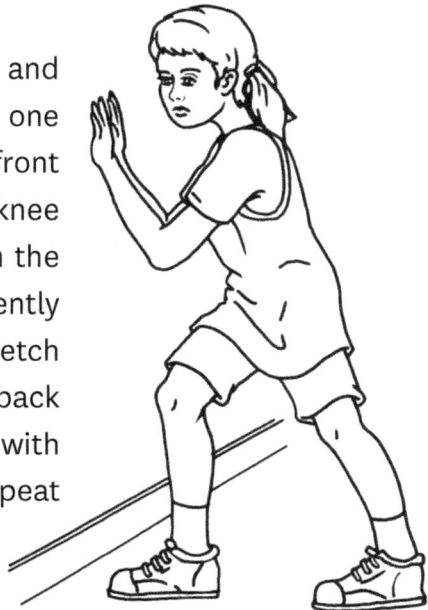

Is basketball your favourite sport?

Do you watch the star players and think …
I wish I could do that?

Well, this is the book for you!

Practise basic basketball skills
at home using this guide
and improve your game.

Maybe you'll be a
basketball star one day!

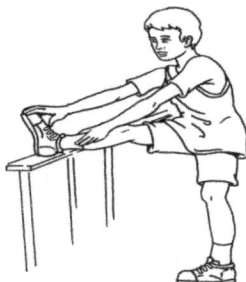

The **Sporting Skills Series** aims to provide useful skills
practice and activities for beginning sports stars.
Other titles are in development.

Garry Powell, is an experienced teacher,
sports trainer and author.

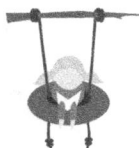

Wellington
books for kids

www.ingramcontent.com/pod-product-compliance
Lightning Source LLC
Chambersburg PA
CBHW032103020426
42335CB00011B/472